FASTING IS THE FOUNDATION

A Real Man's View of Unbelievable Freedom

WRITTEN BY RYAN SMITH

WITH KIM SMITH

An Unbelievable Freedom Book

DEDICATION

When I was a young man, struggling with my weight, my emotions, and my life, I had a very private dream of writing a book about becoming a happy, healthy person, a book that would inspire readers to change their lives. That dream didn't come true until my wife encouraged me to push through my fears and write Unbelievable Freedom. *I dedicate this book to my wife Kimberly. She is my light, my rock, and my biggest supporter. She sees goodness in me that I cannot see in myself. I am eternally grateful.*

The most important kind of freedom is to be what you really are. You trade in your reality for a role. You trade in your sense for an act. You give up your ability to feel, and in exchange, put on a mask. There can't be any large-scale revolution until there's a personal revolution, on an individual level. It's got to happen inside first.

JIM MORRISON

Table of Contents

Welcome From Kim

Greetings!

This is the 9th Unbelievable Freedom Habit Guide I've introduced, and this time, it's with a special kind of excitement. *Fasting Is The Foundation: A Real Man's View of Unbelievable Freedom* is written by my husband, Ryan Smith. It's his second book, a follow up to *Unbelievable Freedom*, the memoir we co-authored in 2018 about our journey with weight. Since that time, he's written extensively, penning dozens of posts for our blog, as well as drafting his first novel. But when I invited him to get involved in this series, he put everything on hold to create this guide based on his own personal practices.

Ryan is a wonderful teacher, writer, and yes, husband! I've always known him as a seeker of truth and freedom. I have watched him strive to achieve health and happiness from day one. When we met, he was in a post-weight loss "honeymoon", and like any honeymoon, he wanted to believe it was all happily-ever-after from there. It turns out, we both did some magical thinking in those early years.

There have been tough times and hard lessons since, but fasting together is what has taught us the most. We engage in it as an intentional, freedom-bringing practice. We show up and live this lifestyle every day, and we continue to reap the rewards.

Because of my starring role in Ryan's story, I can attest that every word in these pages is authentic. I'm so proud of the work he is doing, and I hope you're enriched by what he's shared here.

Enjoy Your Life,
Kim

Introduction

Unbelievable freedom. That's what we all want, right? The freedom to be healthy and strong. The freedom to feel joy and live in the moment. The freedom to love and feel a sense of purpose in the world. For many years, I didn't feel any of that, and I didn't believe that I ever would.

I vividly remember a scene from early childhood that captures one of the last moments of true freedom I would feel for decades. I was about seven years old. My father was a truck driver, and I was fascinated by the various buttons and switches on the big dashboard panel. One day, my father announced he would be dropping me off at school in the big truck. I was so excited. I imagined all the other kids on the playground would be so envious when they saw me climbing down from that enormous machine. I pictured all the kids lining up and pumping their arms up and down, asking for a toot from the horn, and my father would disrupt the whole neighborhood with a long (and completely unnecessary) sonic blast.

It wasn't meant to be. The timing of my arrival at school was off, and when I climbed out of the truck cabin, I realized that none of the busses had arrived yet. There were a couple of other early-arriving kids milling about, and one disgruntled teacher, but no adoring throng rushing forward for a closer look. No blast from the horn, either. My father drove away, and I was left alone on a nearly deserted playground with nothing but my plastic briefcase and crushed expectations. I handled it the only way I knew how as a seven-year-old oddball. I ran. I ran a lot. I raced from one side of the school yard to the other.

In those days, I loved to run. I was skinny and fast. It felt like flying, and I still vaguely remember the sense of outrunning all the swirling thoughts and emotions that were bouncing around in my head. I probably looked like a total weirdo, dashing back and forth like I was being chased by monsters, but I didn't care. I was unbelievably free.

Maybe in another life, I could have used running to process all my negative experiences and become a deliriously happy marathoner. That wasn't meant to be either. I soon discovered that eating food, and lots of it, served a similar, though less healthy, function. I learned to shove down unpleasant emotions, all my sadness, anxiety, loneliness and fears, under candy and potato chips. Within a year or two, I had left my skinny and speedy self behind, replaced by a shy, chubby loner.

I don't know if my confidence eroded because I got fat, or if I got fat to deal with my lack of confidence. It's a classic chicken and the egg situation, but at the end of the day, it doesn't really matter. I gained weight steadily over the years, and with the increase in pounds came a pervasive sense of brokenness. Like Pinnochio, I dreamed of being a real boy. I didn't care about sports, but I wanted to be able to do them like the other kids. I was nervous about a lot of social situations, but I wanted to be included. I was no slave to fashion, but I was aware that Husky pants were not cool. I wanted to feel normal, but I had no idea how to achieve that goal.

By the time I reached middle school, I internalized a lot of stupid rules about masculinity and fat and weight loss. I had to count calories and keep them low to lose weight, but real men eat a ton of food and eat it all with gusto. Gotta keep up your strength and build that muscle! The only exercise that will burn fat is aerobics, but aerobics classes are all about spandex and sparkles. Real men play sports, damn it! But wait. I hated sports. It was all very confusing and contradictory.

When I first tried to lose weight in my teens, I didn't know where to turn for answers. It was the era of the TV infomercial, and that market was dominated by women. Some were more knowledgeable than others, but most seemed more about selling colorful workout clothes than solid weight loss plans. I tried some of those products out of ignorant desperation.

Who remembers the classic "step aerobics" workouts that were so popular in the 80's? I tried them because they promised to raise my heart rate to the "fat burning zone", as long as I was replacing all fat in my diet with Snackwell cookies and fat free cheese, of course. I spent many days jumping around the living room trying to keep up with a group of women who were already thin and fit, grinning like circus clowns and offering lame advice like "C'mon, girls, feel the burn". Oh, I felt the burn, all right, usually as a tendon lost contact with the bone.

Sigh. It wasn't a good fit. Where was the sweaty, fat guy rolling his eyes and muttering sarcastic comments? I wanted someone I could relate to, someone who understood the limitations of my body in its current state, someone who could offer sound advice that didn't require dance lessons.

American capitalism being what it is, more programs for men began to materialize, but I struggled with those, too. All the guys in those videos were fitness-model types, Greek Gods in short shorts and Nikes. I preferred them to Aquanet and sparkles, but they were unattainable wish fulfillment. I wanted to **be** those guys, but I knew in my heart that genetics were not on my side. No amount of weight lifting was going to transform me into the Diet Coke guy. It also turns out that drinking gallons of Diet Coke won't work either. Who knew???

As I reached adulthood and my issues with weight became more serious, I knew what I wanted. I wanted to eat and live like a real person. I wanted to be physically active and strong, so I could do real things, like hike and bike and play with dogs. I wanted to be healthy and to learn how to take care of myself so I could age gracefully, avoid diseases of excess and be a proper example for my children. Sure, it would be nice to look like a celebrity, but that was no longer the point.

It took years of searching, experimenting and failing, but I've finally found the answer with Gin Stephens' *Delay Don't Deny*. Intermittent fasting is the real deal, guys. I eat what I want. I don't have to shun anything. I don't have to sit on the sidelines of any barbeque, birthday party or holiday. I don't have to eat like a bird. I don't have to pretend that I don't LOVE food. I eat with enthusiasm and make no apologies.

IF also made me realize that exercise for its own sake is not really necessary. When you eat is far more important than working out for fat loss. Movement is awesome and promotes good overall health, but gone are the days of jumping around in a contrived routine. Now I walk a lot, sometimes I run, I do yoga, and maybe someday I will climb a real mountain. Whatever I do, it will be living my life, not "doing a workout".

My wife Kim and I started intermittent fasting together, and she also lost extra weight and reclaimed her health. We were thrilled to realize that IF not only addressed the physical aspects of weight loss, but it created space to address long-standing emotional and spiritual issues as well. We became healthier *and* happier. We were so excited about the changes in our lives that we wrote a memoir about our journey. Because of the freedom we felt, we called it....you guessed it.... *Unbelievable Freedom: How We Transformed Our Health and Happiness with Intermittent Fasting.*

I've now been in weight loss maintenance for two years, and the benefits of intermittent fasting have continued to deepen. That's the reason for this book. I've realized that my fasting practice has opened the door for a number of other practices in my life that finally tackle the reasons I gained weight in the first place. I still struggle in my life, as we all do, but I also recognize the joy of progress over perfection. Fasting is my foundation for Unbelievable Freedom.

How to Use This Book

One of my greatest struggles in life has been the pursuit of perfection over practice. It's the root of so many failures, not only in the area of diet and exercise, but in all aspects of my life. I often felt stuck. If I can't do something right the first time, isn't it better to just not try? It was an attempt to protect myself from disappointment and hurt, but it caused more pain by keeping me too comfortable to grow and feel and change.

This workbook shares my experience with intermittent fasting as a foundation, yes, but focuses on how IF gave me a new perspective on my entire life, allowing me to develop practices that moved beyond weight loss.

There are five major sections in this book. FOOD, MOVEMENT, MOOD, LOVE, and PURPOSE. Each section will describe my journey to new thinking around that topic. I'll also share my top three practices in each section. These practices are not goals or prescriptions. For me, it's not about perfection or finish lines. Rather I'm striving to embrace ways of being that allow me to reflect and improve and feel more joy.

I've also included some questions to process each practice. Not as assignments or mandates, but as prompts to help you think about how you can implement small practices in your own life that can lead to big and unexpected dividends.

Enjoy the journey.

Diets work...until they don't

I spent many years on the diet roller coaster, looking for the elusive *answer*, the one definitive way of eating and exercising that would solve all my problems and not only make me thin, but happy and healthy and taller and better looking. You get the idea. I was putting a lot of expectations on this mysterious answer.

There was no shortage of people looking to provide the solution either. Bookstores and the internet are full of products all making similar claims. I think I tried them all. I counted calories, eliminated fat in my diet, eliminated carbs in my diet, eliminated fun in my diet. I tried Atkins and The Zone, South Beach and the Carbohydrate Addict's Diet. All of my attempts were characterized by a sense of desperate optimism. This time will be THE time that I take off the weight and everything falls into place.

Nope. Each diet followed the pattern of a bad relationship. There was the flirtation and excitement of something new, when the future was bright and hopeful. This was followed by the honeymoon phase, when all the bad foods hit the trash can like love letters from an old girlfriend and were replaced by tub of low fat cottage cheese or celery sticks or fatty cuts of beef. Whatever. I rearranged my whole life to make room for the diet. This was forever, after all. Then the first cracks in the veneer. A slip up. A cheat. The messy breakup. Repeat.

Sometimes this cycle played out over a few weeks. Sometimes a few days. Sometimes it started at breakfast yet crashed and burned by lunch. Yet I continued the search and repeated the effort. Over and over and over again. When I look back on those years now, I'm not sure how I persevered. I was driven by an unwavering sense that if thin and healthy people existed, and they did, I saw them every day, then there must be a way to become one of them. I just had to find it.

I had two serious relationships with ways of eating that were more successful. When I was 29 years old, I was diagnosed with diabetes. That scared me and motivated me to make some major changes in my life. I decided to indulge my longtime curiosity with vegetarianism and leapt into a full-blown love affair with it. I ate massive quantities of fruit and veggies, rice and beans, meat substitutes, and low-fat pasta or bread. I loved being a vegetarian and it seemed to really work for me...for about two years. I lost 120 pounds and brought my diabetes into tight control. I loudly and proudly proclaimed that I found "the one" I had been seeking for so long.

It wasn't meant to be. The beginning of the end was the occasional cheat. A little junk food here. A little more dessert there. I remember the day I decided to go to Wendy's and eat a cheeseburger. I framed it as a conscious choice, but it was really an abandonment of something that wasn't really working as well as I claimed it was. I let it all go and regained all the weight and then some.

My second long-term relationship with a diet plan came a few years later, again triggered by a health crisis. My blood sugar was higher than ever, and I needed to make a change to avoid serious consequences. This time, the Paleo diet seemed like a brilliant choice. It was basically the opposite of being a vegetarian and look how that turned out. I shunned carbs like bread, pasta, and rice but ate copious amounts of veggies, meat, and fat. I lost those same 120 pounds eating this way. My diabetes was again under control. I shouted to the hills that I had finally found the answer! Does this sound familiar to you? It did to me, too, but I didn't truly see it for what it was.

The entire pattern repeated itself. My Christmas treats became New Year's treats became Valentine's treats. My habits unraveled and the weight started coming back like a freight train. I regained 40 pounds and probably would have gained much more if I hadn't finally interrupted the dysfunctional relationships with food: this time with intermittent fasting.

Intermittent fasting taught me a critically important lesson. Diets work...until they don't. I lost a lot of weight with diametrically opposed ways of eating, but I couldn't maintain it for the long haul. Why? I think I was expecting too much. I wasn't eating to fuel my body or to achieve better health or to enjoy my life. I was eating to "make up" for a lifetime of being fat. If I'm being honest, I was probably punishing myself a bit, too. How dare I eat a cupcake if I had so much weight to lose? Living by rigid dietary rules was the cross I had to bear because my mind and body were broken and had to be fixed by a prescription.

Fasting is different because it's not a diet at all. It's a strategy, a bio hack, a habit, *a practice*. It's not an identity that I must hold up and proclaim to the world. A few years back, I flirted with the concept of a zero carb diet, essentially eating nothing but meat and fat. I read up on it online and was growing enamored by the diet until I read one person's strategy about how to deal with attending a wedding reception. This proponent of zero carb suggested bringing cooked chicken breasts in a cooler and going out to the car to eat them while the meal was served. It was presented as a badge of honor, a declaration of commitment to health, a resolve to give a huge middle finger to society saying happiness and cake are synonymous. That appealed to me in a major way.

But...I imagined myself standing outside eating boiled chicken out of the trunk of my car, the muffled sounds of laughter and tinkling silverware from inside where the guests enjoyed a delicious meal and wedding cake. It didn't feel like a solution to me, just substituting one struggle for another.

These days, I don't say 'never' about any food. I don't have to. I eat the way people eat when they've had a problem with weight in the first place. I eat a variety of foods. I go to the BBQ or the party or faculty potluck and eat like a person. The difference lies in **when** I eat instead of **what** I eat. It feels like food freedom, and the following practices will show you what that looks like.

Practice 1 - Eat what you want not what you should

One of the biggest problems with diets is this: diets are all about telling us what to do. Eat this. Don't eat that. Like there's a one-size-fits-all formula for the specific foods humans are designed to eat. But people aren't wired like that. Sure, I went out and bought celery sticks because my calorie-counting diet said I could have unlimited amounts of them, but I don't really like celery, so I never ate it for very long.

When I was following Paleo, I was convinced that I *shouldn't* eat carbs, but I like bread, especially in the form of a roll with a juicy hamburger inside. Don't worry if your tastes are narrow or a little weird or don't conform to conventional dietary wisdom. Follow an intermittent fasting protocol and within your eating window, eat the foods you enjoy until you're no longer hungry. It makes sense. As you continue your fasting lifestyle, your preferences will likely change anyway, and you might be surprised to be craving new foods. Just eat what you like, and your body will sort it out.

Practice 2 - Stop restricting and start fueling your life

I spent a lot of time and energy obsessing about calories. If I wasn't actively counting them, I was trying to avoid food I thought was high in calories, or I was force-feeding myself low-calorie food I didn't really want. Sometimes I was counting fat grams or carbs or something else. In any event, the diets I tried always told me to restrict *something*. I was driven by a mindset that insisted I couldn't lose weight unless I was giving something up, cutting something out or feeling denied and deprived. It's not true. Stop restricting and let food be the fuel that gives you the energy to do all the other important things in your life.

You should feel satisfied when you are done eating for the day, so eat a snack if you want to. Eat a delicious, nutritious meal that you love eating. Have a little dessert or something after dinner if you are still hungry. Let go of the fear of food. It's supposed to feel good. If you are feeling persistent hunger pangs or some other unpleasant sensation, it's not a sign that you're burning fat. It's a sign that you need fuel. That's not only OK, it's awesome.

Practice 3 - Separate eating from feeling

The third food-related practice is the trickiest one. I've been in maintenance for a couple of years, and I still work on this one more days than not. That's why it's a practice, something that we apply every day with an eye towards progress, not perfection. Every time I lost weight in the past, I failed to see something that I really needed to face. I was using food to manage my feelings. In fact, I connected food to almost every feeling, good or bad.

Intermittent fasting finally gave me the space to see just how much I was doing that. I generally fast for 20-22 hours per day. That's a lot of time for emotions to well up. Before I would have eaten some chips or candy to push those feelings aside. I didn't even notice I was doing it most of the time. Now the true power is in the noticing. I can see that I'm not really hungry, and I use other activities to deal with a feeling. If I'm bored, I can take my dog for a walk or find an interesting movie to watch. If I'm anxious, I can meditate or work on a writing project. Or sometimes I simply acknowledge that, nope, that's not hunger, that's an emotion, and move on with my day.

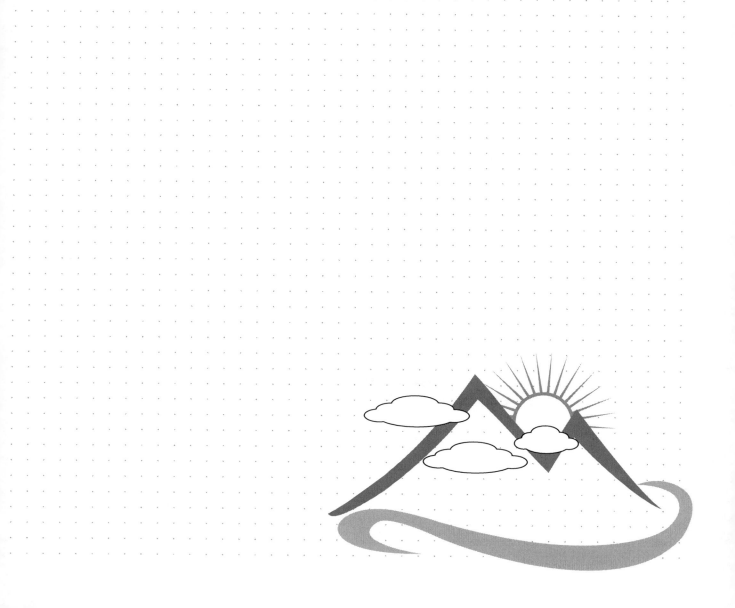

Process

▲ Think about your own current practices around food.

▲ Do you eat foods that you don't really like because you have the idea that you *should* like them?

▲ What do you like to eat?

▲ Do you eat less than you really want to eat because you think you should feel hungry and deprived to lose weight?

▲ Do you think there are bad foods to be avoided?

▲ Are you using food to avoid feeling your emotions?

▲ What are some things you like to do instead of eating when you are feeling happy, stressed, sad or lonely?

Cavemen didn't work out, either

"You play football, right?" I was a teenager the first time someone asked me that question, some well-intentioned adult trying to reconcile the fat kid in front of them with the idea that all boys must love sports. I continued to get the question into adulthood, usually from students who were just curious about what I was like in high school. Intellectually, I knew the question was harmless, nothing more than random conversation, even if it was fueled by false assumptions. I wanted to say, "Nope, just fat", but I resisted that impulse and shrugged it off every time.

Inwardly, the question was a real trigger for me. Our culture is dominated by love of sports, and that love is tangled up in what it means to be a real boy and a real man. As I started gaining weight rapidly around third grade, my already-lackluster interest in sports shriveled completely. As I mentioned before, I loved to run, but it didn't seem like a competition to me, and even that became difficult when I got too heavy to enjoy it. I was painfully aware that I was excluded (or excluded myself) from a lot of activities that the other boys were doing.

This conundrum of wanting to fit in and *be* fit, but having no real interest in doing the things I perceived as necessary, followed me through my teen years and into adulthood. It was the driving force behind every decision to follow one fitness craze after another. I tried aerobics videos marketed to women in a desperate strategy to lose weight, so I could maybe, just maybe, be physically active, or at least *look* like I could be. I did those workouts like a dirty secret, typically in the basement when nobody else was home. I clearly was not the target demographic for those products, and most of them were truly designed for women who were already fit, so it was doomed to fail. Nothing about it worked for me.

The programs designed for men that emerged in the late 80's and early 90's were ultimately no better. I was excited at the prospect of mastering Tae Bo and having a boxer's physique, but I conveniently overlooked the reality of the situation. I had barely moved for over 20 years. Throwing aggressive air punches and jumping from side to side for 30 minutes? Well, I guess it did feel kind of manly, but it also hurt like hell. It cemented what I already "knew". Being healthy and strong was not in the cards for me, and by extension, I would always feel inadequate and less than. The Pinocchio thing all over again.

I was over 40 years old when I finally connected to a fitness philosophy in a way that felt natural to me. I'd received the bad news that my blood sugar was out of control again and started losing weight with a high fat, low carb diet. I was reading Mark Sisson's *Primal Blueprint* and Abel James' *Fat Burning Man* and loving the approach: focus on replicating the way our prehistoric ancestors lived, moving to improve the functionality of the human body. It didn't seem competitive to me, and I saw how it would make my life better. Not a mythical fantasy life when I inexplicably became a fitness model, but a life in which I could rake the leaves without being sore for a week afterwards, or bend over to tie my shoes without risk of a pulled muscle.

When I began fasting, I reintroduced grains and beans and other carbs to my diet, and that briefly distracted me from the tenets of Paleo fitness that I actually liked. I was hung up by all-or-nothing thinking. Can I work out like a caveman if I eat bread later? Do I have to go back to the step aerobics I hated if I let a dessert pass my lips? Then I remembered what I always tell my ninth-grade students about study strategies. You have to do what works for you. There are no hard and fast rules. If flash cards make you crazy, don't use them. Find what works and ditch the rest. If that's true for learning grammar rules, then it could be true for diet and fitness, right?

Yup. These days I fast clean for 18-22 hours per day, then eat what I want and enjoy in my window. I also move like a caveman, focusing on function and fun. I don't "exercise" or "work out" anymore. No more DVD's, canned programs, special programs or machines. Prehistoric man walked a lot, and so do I. It's my favorite way to move. Whenever the weather allows, I go outside for a walk. I don't time myself or set specific goals around it, but my preferred routes tend to be about 3 miles. During my walks, I throw in a hill or a set of steps whenever I can. I no longer maintain exercise journals or logs. That always felt like pressure to me, so I don't do it. I just get out and move.

I started doing yoga a couple years ago, and I still practice every day, mostly with the guidance of *ManFlowYoga* on YouTube. People have been using yoga techniques for thousands of years to improve flexibility and balance, alleviate stress, and build muscle. I was skeptical that yoga could do all of that, but I was wrong. Yoga is awesome. I've become more muscular than I ever thought I could. I have noticeable biceps, and the shadow of abs. My legs are strong and sculpted. I stand up straighter, and I can touch my toes without bending my knees.

Will any of this turn back the clock and make me look like the Diet Coke guy from the 80's? Nope. But I realized that I never really wanted that. I wanted the strength and overall fitness to live a real life. As I write these words, a snowstorm is approaching Maine. I still don't like to shovel snow, but I'm confident I have the strength to do it. I can also go for a hike and not get left behind. I can pick up a toddler without strain, or rearrange the living room furniture, or mow the lawn, or dig a hole to plant a flower. You get the idea. Function and fun. That feels like the freedom of movement, and the following practices will show you more.

Practice 1 - Start small to leave room to grow

Traditional exercise programs didn't work for me because they were so...much. They were high octane, all-in, athletic endeavors. My spirit was willing, but my body just wasn't prepared. I suspect many of those programs were designed by people who were never obese themselves. They were catering to customers' wishful thinking instead of their very real, but not very exciting, needs. If you've been sedentary for a long time or have a lot of extra pounds in the way, start small to leave room for growth. I get it. It will feel like a cop out, like it's not enough, but consider the end game.

The point is improvement and progress, not injury and burnout. If walking to the mailbox is all you can comfortably do right now, then that's all you need to do. Your body will start the work of getting stronger and healthier without sidelining you with aches, pains and regrets. Tomorrow, go to the corner. I'm not sure why it took me so long to learn this lesson, but it sure did. In other areas of our lives, we recognize this. Ever teach a kid to clean his room? How about building a snowman? Starting small to end strong is a commonsense approach to almost anything. It might trigger some feelings of impatience, but in the end, it's the key to staying in the game.

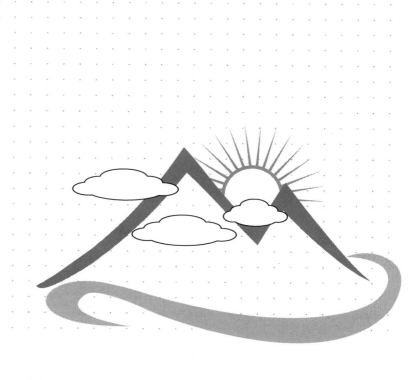

Practice 2 - Move to get things done or feel like fun

If you're anything like me, you have an aversion to wasting time. I was convinced that an hour-long workout was *necessary* but it didn't feel like fun to me, and it didn't feel all that productive either. I endured it, then went about my business. I wonder how many times I suffered through an exercise routine, then felt tired and worn out while mowing my lawn or cleaning out the garage. I would've been better off just doing the chores, but I thought I had to get my fitness in first. All movement is good. It counts!

As I move into my third year of weight loss maintenance at 47 years old, I'm finally getting better every year, and I never "exercise on purpose". Do things that get things done or feel like fun, just like the cavemen did. Walking and stretching are fun for me. Sports not so much, but who knows? Maybe one of these days I will start running again like when I was a kid. Or join a disc frisbee team. If it feels fun or gets something done, I'll do it and improve my health while I'm at it. Instead of working out like you *should*, think about what you actually like to do and do that.

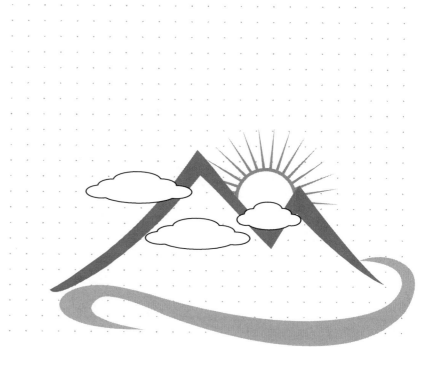

Practice 3 - Let fitness happen while you're focusing on the big picture

When I was obese and trying to take action to change that, I was always in such a hurry. I would look for obvious signs of progress before any progress could realistically be attained. Have you ever hopped on a scale minutes after a workout expecting to see pounds lost? Or inspected your profile in a mirror after one day of clean eating? I ate kale, why am I not thinner, damn it?!!?! It just doesn't work like that. We mistakenly make the pursuit of a healthier life into the sum total of our lives. We stare at it and study it and agonize about it, forgetting to really live in the meantime. Let fitness happen while you're focusing on the big picture of your life. You will make gains when you are not looking so closely.

Ever watch a huge snowbank melt away in the spring? Me neither. We vaguely notice the change over time, then marvel when we see bare earth again. Yoga was like for me. I just did it every day because I liked it, and it felt good. At some point, my wife remarked that my body was feeling so much leaner and more powerful, and, yes, it was true. Find the activities you like to do, do them, and get on with your life. You don't need to constantly measure it, clock it, or chart it. Just let it happen and enjoy the results.

Process

▲ Consider your own current practices around movement.

▲ Are you working out in ways that don't feel good, or maybe even make you sore, uncomfortable or injured?

▲ Are you pushing yourself too hard too fast to get results now?

▲ Do you hold on to belief systems about what you *should* do, even if you don't want to?

▲ What kind of movement do you need to get things done in your life?

▲ What do you like to do for fun?

▲ Are there areas of your life that you neglect because you're spending too much time focusing on fitness?

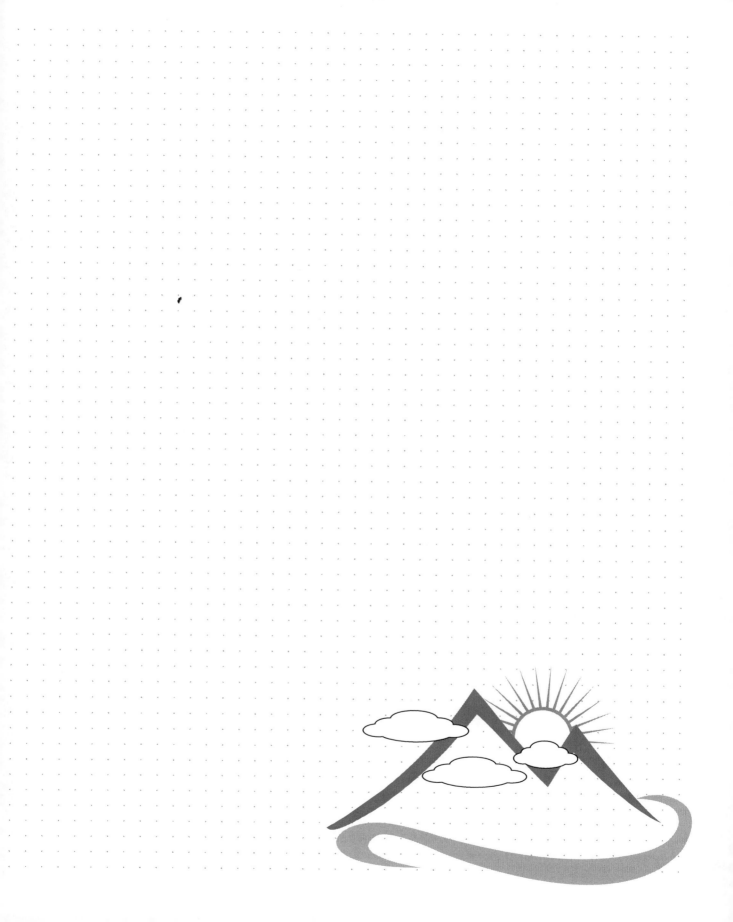

Happiness is real...but it doesn't just happen

This section of the book is the hardest one for me to write, but I decided to put it right in the middle because I think it's the beating heart of my fasting practice. It represents the most important realizations I've had about gaining and losing weight, and even more significantly, what it will take for me to remain in maintenance for the rest of my life.

When I pass back graded essays to my students, I often ask them, "Do you want the good news or the bad news first"? They generally want the good news first. Who doesn't want to delay a bummer for as long as possible? You did a great job on your introductions. Awesome! But the transitions in the body paragraphs? Well, we're not quite there yet. Let's practice some more.

Inevitably, there are elements of good and bad news in most situations, right? Intermittent fasting and weight loss is no exception. When I was obese, I desperately believed that if I could just lose the weight, I would be happy. I had grand visions of being thin and healthy, muscular and attractive. Once I attained a certain number on the scale, I would be excited about life. I would become insanely popular, and everyone would clamor to spend time with me. My days would be fun-filled with trips and parties and passions and laughter. I would be funnier, more confident, more competent and more alive.

I probably should have realized that losing weight, even 120 pounds, would not completely re-wire my brain and make me a whole new person. But as silly as it sounds, I didn't really get it. I held on to that belief like a life preserver because ultimately, I wanted to better in ways that transcended my size, but I had no idea how to do it. On some level, I must have suspected the truth. That's probably why so many diets ended in failure. If I lost the weight and still wasn't happy, then game over. As long as I was fat and trying, then I could cling to the hope that it could be different.

So, the good news? Happiness is real. The bad news? It doesn't just happen. When I lost 120 pounds on a vegetarian diet and again years later with a Paleo diet, I didn't do much to address my mental health. I expected to be happy, and when I wasn't, I started to make choices that sent me back to the starting gate. I struggled with unresolved depression and anxiety, and in the absence of food to self-medicate those feelings, I was white knuckling through my days and eventually sabotaged my weight loss. Repeat the cycle.

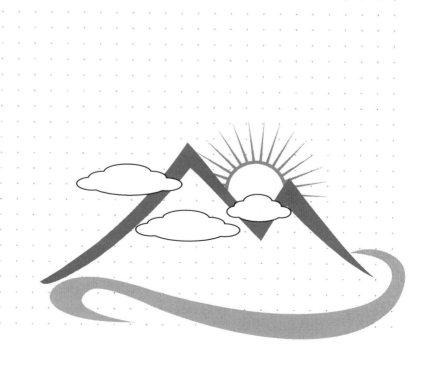

Don't get me wrong. I was happier than I had been before. I was proud of my accomplishment and felt more comfortable in my own skin. I was definitely more confident, and dynamics with the people in my life shifted as I acted more like my true self. But my lifelong issues with managing my mood and emotions didn't magically disappear. I still isolated myself from intense social situations. I retreated from powerful emotions, even with (and maybe especially with) the people I love the most. If I had accepted that the real work was just beginning, I could have rewritten some patterns earlier, but I wasn't ready to do it. I judged myself instead and that led me backwards.

The discovery of intermittent fasting was a powerful turning point in my life. So powerful that I hesitate to type the next words in case someone misunderstands me and stops reading, but it's the truth, so here goes. Fasting is awesome. It can reset your metabolism and reshape your body. It can show you what hunger really is and teach you to eat to appetite. It allows you to eat like a real person and even become an intuitive eater, who doesn't eat just because.

But...intermittent fasting is not the finish line. It's not a miracle cure for every struggle in your life. Even if you lose a ton of weight, you will still be you, and it will take more work to achieve the happiness you wanted weight loss to bring. I went through a year-long honeymoon phase where I thought all my problems were solved, but it wasn't the case. I gradually became aware that not only did my feelings of depression and anxiety still exist, they were welling up more than ever, and I wasn't using junk food to deal with them. It was a runaway train picking up steam.

I could have easily jumped back on the rollercoaster and tossed IF on the heap of things I'd tried and angrily discarded, but it's so different this time. *Intermittent fasting is different.* The "magic" of the fast is not that it unpacked all the emotional baggage, but that it finally gave me the space and clarity to really see the problem for what it is. OH!!! You got fat because you were a sad, lonely, scared little kid and didn't know what to do about it. Gaining weight was never a character defect, it was a brave (though misguided) attempt to survive and thrive. It's kind of hopeful, really!

I spend a lot of time in online communities for intermittent fasters. I see so many people in the place I used to be in, cautiously optimistic about IF as a ``new diet". Some of them seem to have similar emotional struggles. As they ask questions about what kinds of foods they are "allowed" to eat, or if it's "OK" that they ate a piece of cake at a birthday party, I want them to know that diet thinking can soon be a thing of the past. It's possible to be unbelievably free of that, but I also want to affirm that it's the trajectory that many of us need to take.

I always suspected that being depressed and anxious *might* be the real root of my discontent, but I didn't want to hear it. I couldn't really care about emotional and spiritual growth when my damned pants were cutting off my circulation. Once the physical aspect of weight loss was behind me, I was ready to tackle the underlying work. It's hard and messy and ongoing. I'm a work in progress with many miles to go, but light at the end of the end of this tunnel burns so much brighter with fasting as my foundation.

I use the following three practices to feel the freedom of emotional balance and true happiness.

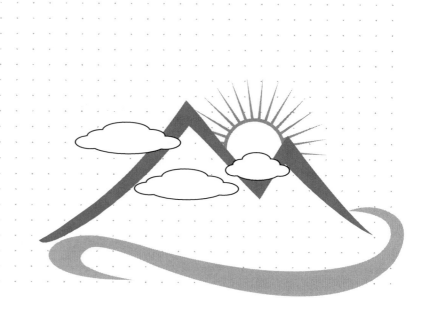

Practice 1 - Reconnect to the things you loved when you were a kid

As a little kid, I loved two things more than anything else. Superheroes and Stephen King. I was a comic book reading, Saturday morning cartoon watching, nose buried in a book little nerd. I lived for those experiences. Every week was a countdown to the latest episode of *Spiderman and his Amazing Friends* or *The Kids' Super Power Hour with Shazam* (yes, that was a real thing). I felt a powerful affinity for the mild mannered alter ego who could transform into something amazing. Stephen King's book *Carrie* is hands down my favorite book of all time. I read it for the first time when I was about eleven. It lit me up. A screwed up kid who is like an alien in the world with the power to knock a house over with *her mind??!!?* Sign me up, please!

In retrospect, I see that I was drawn to ideas and themes pulled directly from my own reality, but at the time, I only knew that I absolutely loved those stories. Reconnect to the things you loved when you were a kid. That kind of love and excitement does not die, but it can get buried under layers of real life. Dig it all back out and feel the best parts of being a kid again. For many of us, memories of childhood became colored by our focus on the negative things, but take the time to rediscover the things that were pure magic.

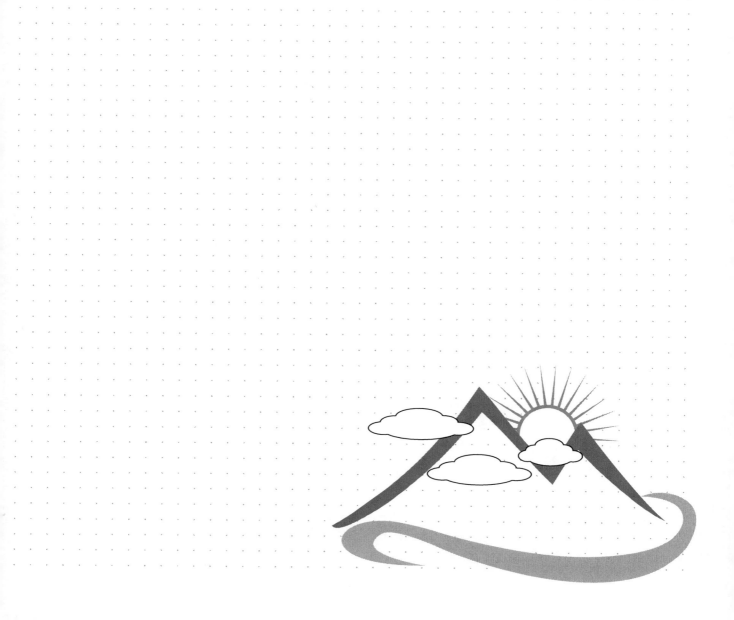

Practice 2 - Do the day you're on

They say that depression is essentially looking backwards with regret, while anxiety is looking forward with fear. As fasting became habitual and my inner thoughts became more clear, this concept hit me like a thunderbolt. I totally do that! I sometimes catch myself replaying an awkward or painful memory from 35 years ago. When I finally pull myself out of the memory, I realize my entire body is experiencing the feeling from the event all over again. I can also spend an entire commute anticipating a tense conversation or argument that hasn't even happened yet, sometimes with such vivid detail that I actually feel scared or resentful or rageful. Did I mention that this thing hasn't even happened in reality?

I used to tell myself that I was just "processing", but I was really programming myself to feel depressed or anxious about things I cannot control. Do the day you're on. Focus on the moments you're truly in. Most of the time being "in the moment" is a pretty safe, even joyful, place to be. I wish it were easier to explain exactly how to do this, but like all the other things I'm realizing about my life, doing the day you're on is about the practice and embracing all the blurry edges. These days when I find myself in the mental time machine, I gently remind myself to return to the present. Some days I have to do that a hundred times, but it's slowly and surely releasing unnecessary emotions that don't serve me.

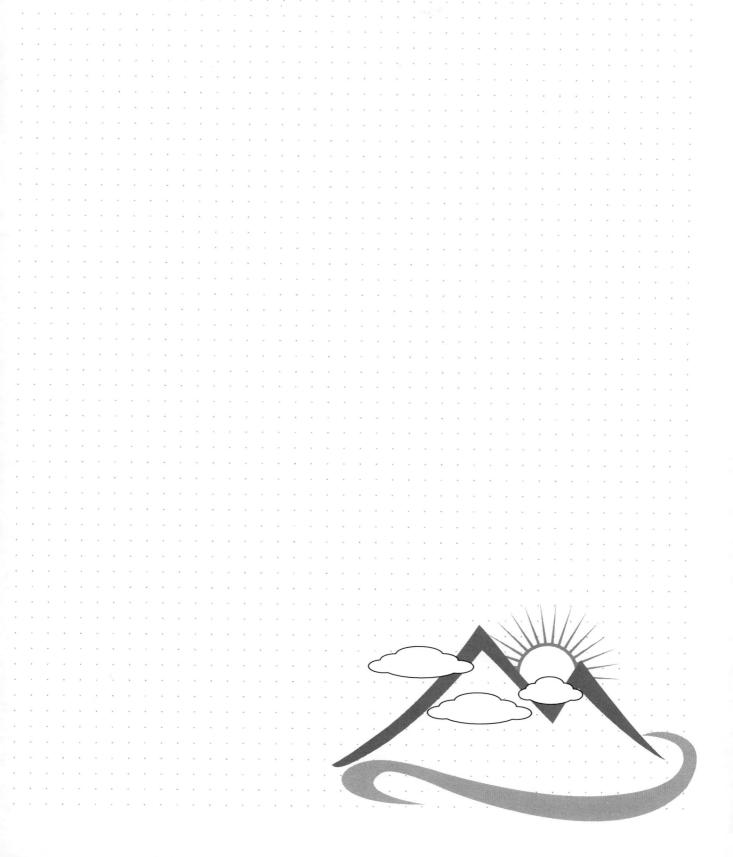

Practice 3 - Get comfortable in your own head

Think about all the ways we try to distract ourselves from the feelings, thoughts, obsessions, memories, and stories about ourselves that swirl around in our brains. Food has been my distraction of choice for much of my life, but there are many others. Television. Music. Mindless internet searches. Facebook scrolling. The endless noise of the modern world combined with my own runaway thought patterns turned my inner landscape into a nearly 24/7 pinball machine, so much clicking, banging, jangling and clacking. Sometimes I wake up to song lyrics playing on a loop in my head, or mindlessly reviewing the plot lines of *The Walking Dead*. What purpose does that serve beyond a constant need to distance myself from just...being?

Get comfortable in your own head. Fasting has helped me to develop this practice by giving me the opportunity to really dial into the cacophony and see that those random thoughts are not really me. I started using guided meditation first thing in the morning. I also consciously choose to sit in silence when I have my morning black coffee instead of filling my head up with news headlines, weather reports or random YouTube videos. I'm slowly learning that all those thoughts come and go, and it's OK.

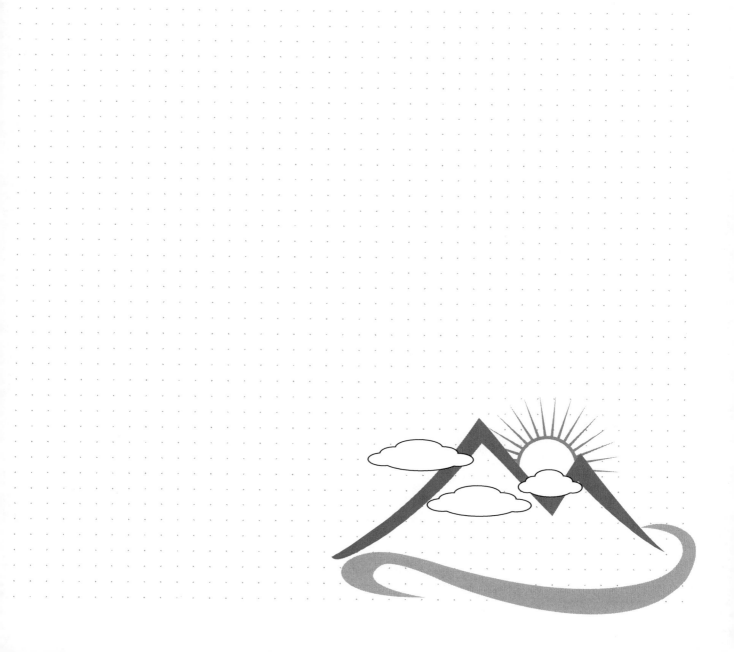

Process

▲ Are you holding onto the idea that losing weight will make you happy?

▲ Do you have other work to do beyond the physical process of losing fat?

▲ What did you love as a child, and how can you bring that feeling back into your life now?

▲ Do you spend too much time in the past or in the future?

▲ How can you spend more of your time in the here-and-now?

▲ Are you distracted by mental clutter?

▲ Have you considered what would happen if you stopped listening to the distractions and embraced silence?

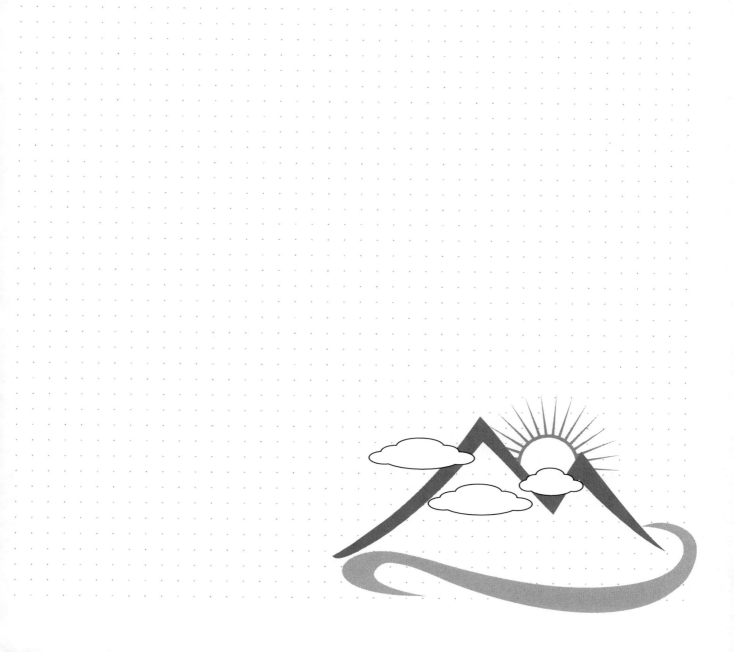

Don't measure yourself with another man's ruler

Intermittent fasting has yielded many unexpected results in my life, but I started fasting for one reason. I wanted to lose weight in a way that would stick. I wanted to look better and feel better. I really just wanted to change my relationship with my pants, so imagine my surprise when fasting changed my relationship with the most important person in my life.

Kim and I talked about our weight loss story in our first book *Unbelievable Freedom*. We wrote the book after our first year of fasting, when everything was flowing and easy and exciting. We were united in a new, common goal to share IF with other people in online communities and our real lives. For the first time in our marriage, we were eating the same meals and preparing them together. We were more energized, active, and, yes, for all the people who wondered but only hinted, the sex *did* get better. The honeymoon phase of fasting ushered in a honeymoon phase for our marriage.

Unfortunately, honeymoon phases, at least in the romantic way we are conditioned to think of them, do not last. We underestimated how much our entire lives would be impacted by the huge change in our eating habits. We gained a LOT of weight together, and even though that was not a healthy emotional strategy, it worked pretty well for a time. We were overeating partners in crime, each enabling the other to eat more and more. On one hand, we were having a great time, going out on Sunday mornings for Egg McMuffin and Dunkin Donut binges, but on the other hand, we were using the food and the excess weight gain to bury emotional realities.

As we reached weight loss maintenance, those emotional realities came back and started causing trouble again. If I ever write a whole book about marriage, I should call it **Love** *is the Foundation* because that's always been true for us. Through all the ups and downs over the past 17 years, the trials of raising children in a shared custody situation, dealing with extended family, money woes, pets and job stress, the weight gains and losses, we have never lost sight of the fact that we love each other madly. We're best friends and soulmates. But just as we know that our foundation is rock solid, we also know the whole house can come crashing down if we don't work to weather the storms together.

Through the process of fasting, specifically learning to feel emotions and cope with them without using food as avoidance, I've learned an important lesson that continues to improve my relationship with my wife. Don't measure yourself with another man's ruler. Just stop with all the expectations and rules about how it's all supposed to be. It just distracts from the beauty of what is.

It's a lesson that Kim and I lived by in some ways since the very beginning. We met in a graduate school class in the spring of 2003. We went on our first date in April, moved in together in August and married in December. That was so unlike me to move so quickly and not sabotage it with overthinking, but some intuition in me said go for it. Ignore all the rational reasons why that was risky and ill-advised. Defy the expectations and just follow my heart. I'm so grateful that I did that.

But over the years, I struggled with all kinds of limiting beliefs about what kind of man and husband I should be, all fueled by unrealistic expectations. I *should* be able to fix everything that goes wrong in my house. I *should* be able to handle every situation with an even temper. I *should* always know the right thing to say and do. Those demands I was placing on myself never served my marriage well.

In my effort to be a good husband, I made Kim's happiness the focal point of my identity. I was paying zero attention to my own emotional baggage and how that was *really* affecting our relationship. In an interesting twist, we realized that Kim was doing the same thing towards me. It was like each of us was trying to parent the other through self-sacrifice. We were avoiding dealing with our own dysfunctional narratives by constantly trying to rewrite the other person's story. We were doing it out of real love, but we were creating the opposite result of what we intended.

With fasting as a foundation, we finally see our emotional issues clearly and we're working through them for the first time. We're doing the real work, and it's making our marriage seem less like work than ever before. The renewed clarity gives us the space to move forward as a team instead of being each other's cheerleader, then fading into the background individually. Of course, we're still each other's biggest fan, but we're also better at getting out of our own way to be better partners.

We now strive for freedom from expectations, and the following three practices will show you how our marriage has grown as a result.

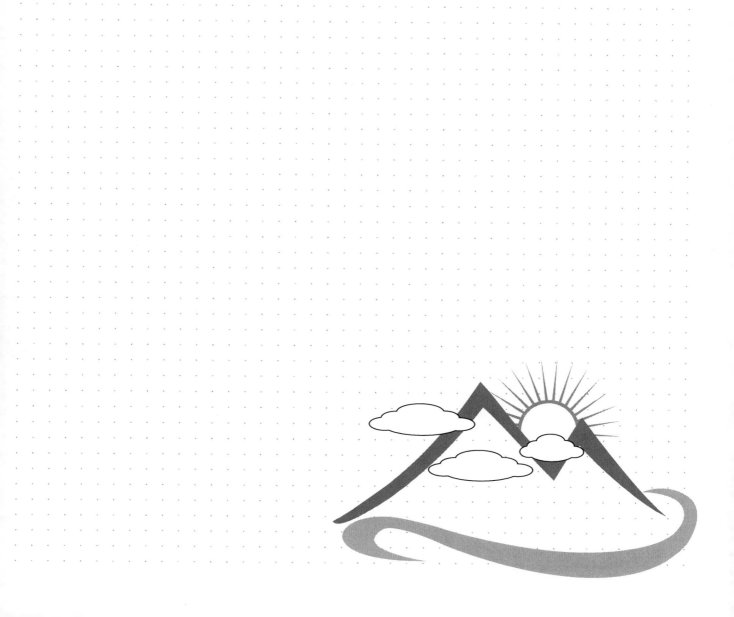

Practice 1 - Reject the rom-com conventions

A recurring theme of our fasting journey has been the realization that much of what we're conditioned to believe is complete and utter garbage. Our expectations around love and marriage are particularly destructive. Romantic comedies are great entertainment, but they really mess with your head. The movie *Pretty Woman* was a huge hit when I was a senior in high school. I may not have been the target demographic, but I loved the story. Hooker with a heart of gold finds true love with charming but lonely corporate raider. Good stuff. Ever wonder why nobody bothered to make *Pretty Woman 2?* The original ends with happily ever after, and that's what we all want. Nobody really wants to see Richard Gere and Julia Robers pack on the pounds and argue about money.

Reject the rom-com conventions. Real love is messy and hard and awesome and beautiful. I think the romance of marriage is in the details that the movies leave out. The other day I mentioned needing a second yoga block for a new sequence I wanted to try. When I got home from a long work day, there was a new yoga block on the dining room table. The knowledge that Kim thought of me and did a little something just to please me is more romantic than any fire escape declaration of love on the big screen. Put more emphasis on small gestures of gratitude than grand ones. That's real love.

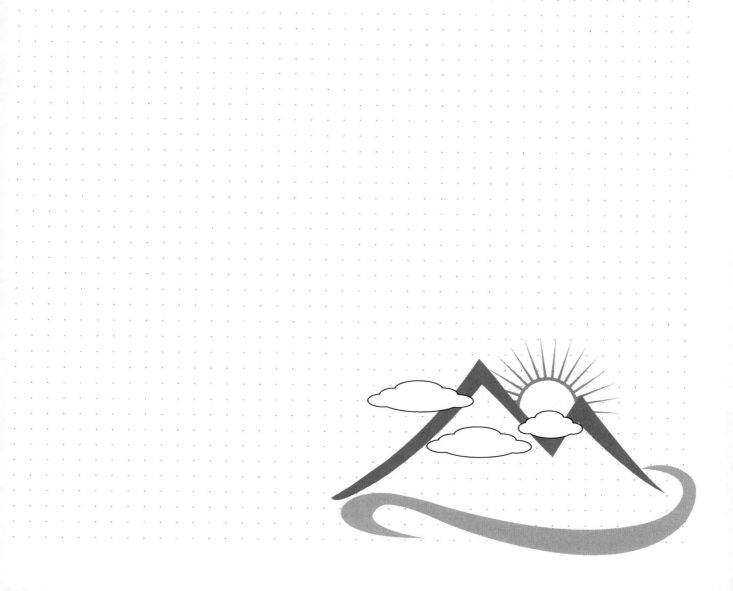

Practice 2 - Balance words and deeds

I'm a fixer. It's a blessing and a curse. If Kim tells me about something that is bothering her, my first impulse is to suggest how to fix the problem, even if she's not really asking for that. I mean well, but I recognize that it's not always the best approach. I show my love and appreciation for people by *doing something.* I will clean the snow off the car and warm it up. I will move the furniture when guests are coming over for a Christmas gathering. I will look for the missing keys. It's my way of saying 'I love you and want to make your life better.'

Balance words and deeds. Doing things for other people is great, but sometimes it can be a way of avoiding saying the things that might be awkward or difficult to say. I'm working more actively on using words to let people know what I'm really feeling. My fasting practice has given me greater insight into my own hardwiring and also helped me see others more clearly. Some people are doers and some are talkers, but most need a balance of both to feel truly loved.

Practice 3 - Focus on the things you love
instead of the things you don't

It's so easy to notice and fixate on the quirks that frustrate us and ignore the countless things we love about another person. This practice reminds me of the first one in the food section of this workbook, eat what you want, not what you *should*. Both practices are about what we choose to focus on, and what we focus on is the thing that grows and looms largest in our minds. If you don't like carrots, you don't have to think about them ever again. Not when there are brussel sprouts and chocolate cake and chicken marsala and biscuits with butter and roasted chickpeas.

Focus on the things that you love instead of the things you don't. Kim has a habit of leaving earrings and necklaces around the house. The window sill. The lazy susan in the center of the dining room table. It drives me nuts. It's OK. She already knows. Fasting makes it easier to focus on the things that are really important. Earrings don't matter in light of the amazing things Kim does for me. She supports me and takes care of me and tells me I'm handsome every day. She has beautiful blue eyes that I notice every single time I look at her...even if I don't say always say it. There's too many things I love about her to worry too much about the other stuff.

Process

▲ Do you have romantic notions about love and marriage that are making you unhappy in your relationship?

▲ Are you comparing your own life to someone else's and worrying that you aren't measuring up?

▲ Do you recognize the way you tend to show your love for other people?

▲ Is it different from your partner's?

▲ How does this cause friction in the relationship?

▲ Do you focus on things that annoy you more than the things that delight you?

▲ What would happen if you changed your approach?

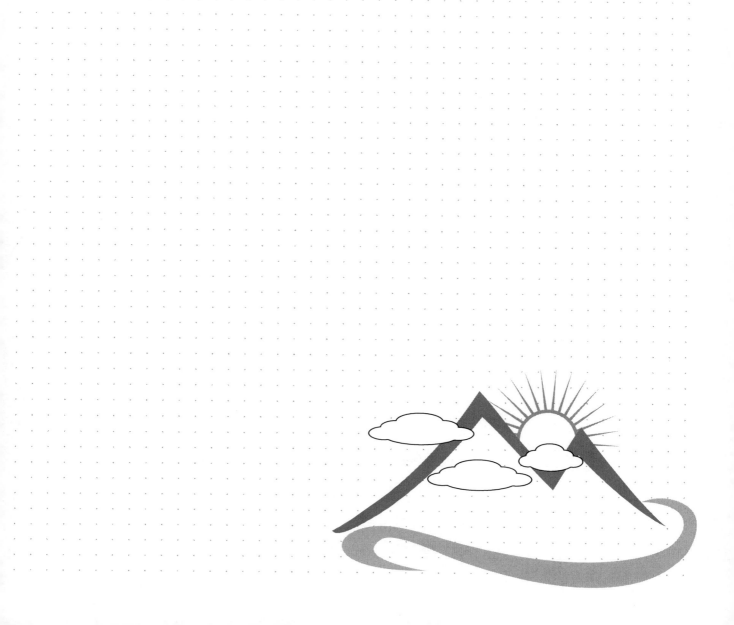

The search for meaning doesn't have a finish line

I've always spent a lot of time in my own head, contemplating big questions. It's why I loved comic books and Stephen King when I was a kid. Some people see those stories as silly kid stuff, but even when I was a kid, I saw something much more significant. Fantasy and science fiction ask us to consider that there are things in the world that are very real, even if we can't see them. We step into the narrative and believe there are limitless possibilities. In those worlds, we always know there's *something more*, even if we can't know for certain what that something is.

As odd as this might sound, reading comic books made me wonder about the greatest mystery there is. Why are we here? What's the point? What is *my* purpose?

For most of my life, I was uncomfortable with the not knowing even though I constantly flirted with the questions. I wanted to believe that every person was created for a special reason, but I was completely turned off by people who claimed to be certain of the answer. The books and stories I loved as a kid managed to balance this inner conflict. My favorite superheroes had a mission that guided them. They were here for a purpose, and they knew what it was, but they lived in a world where Greek gods were real and even death was an enemy that could be vanquished. The messiness of that contradiction was frustrating and thrilling at the same time.

It's the reason I became a teacher. What could be better than getting paid to help kids find meaning in reading and writing? To guide students through the process of forming and answering their own big questions? I learn as much about life from Atticus Finch as I do from Spiderman, and the puzzled expressions on kids' faces when I suggest such a thing? Well, that's pure gold.

Even though I loved teaching, it became just a job as I struggled more with my weight and emotional health. I gave the best of myself to my students for a long time, especially before I met my wife, and I had very little left over for myself. In recent years, after taking off the weight and starting looking at my life in a whole new way, I've realized that teaching is my purpose. It's why I'm here.

I get annoyed with student misbehavior. I sometimes complain bitterly about bureaucracy and budgets. I still shoot a dirty look at the ceiling every time the intercom interrupts my lesson about topic sentences. I suspect that snow days are the universe's way of messing up a carefully-constructed unit. But I also know that teaching connects me to something bigger than myself. There is a powerful magic in a room full of students all thinking, talking, laughing and chewing on an idea at the same time. You can feel it in the air, and it can't be explained by brain chemistry or behavioral science alone.

I think it's a God thing, though I don't know if that's the right word, and I'm OK with that. I don't feel the same need for black and white answers anymore. I am hardwired with a desire for order and clarity, but in this area of life, I'm surprisingly good with the gray. I can't claim to know what will happen when I die, but I do know that every day I'm connected to "something eternal", as the Stage Manager in *Our Town* says. I can't prove it or completely explain it, but I feel it when 20 ninth graders file out of my classroom wishing me a Merry Christmas on the last day before vacation. I feel it when they look to me for guidance when the fire alarm goes off. I feel it when the faces light up when they finally understand something they didn't get before.

Being a teacher and being a student are two sides of the same coin, and in the last few years of my fasting journey, I have learned one thing above all other things. The search for meaning doesn't have a finish line. Diets failed for me because I wanted to find the one true solution, so I could just do that thing and never have to think for myself or change again. Developing my own intuition about what to eat seemed too messy and complicated. I made the same mistake about other parts of life, too, failing to appreciate the best things in life because I couldn't confidently explain them. I don't need to do that anymore.

This feels like freedom to me. The following three practices will show you how I apply this realization in my daily life.

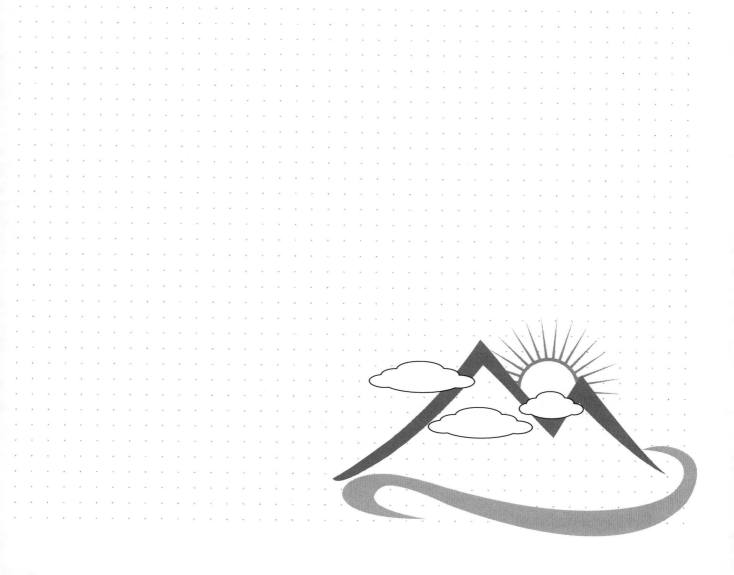

Practice 1 - Acknowledge that life is sometimes bad, and that makes it good

Black and white thinking about the world caused me to waste a lot of time. I abandoned so many things whenever the slightest misstep meant it wasn't perfect. I believed that if something was difficult or ambiguous, it was a sign that I should just not bother. If I ate one bite of cake on the first day of a new diet, I would eat the whole damned thing and start a new diet another day. If I started writing a short story, I would rip it up the first sign of struggle. It was all or nothing.

Acknowledge that life is *sometimes* bad, and that makes it good. I try to live this philosophy in my classroom, which is a little microcosm for life. It's not uncommon to have negative interactions with students, but it's very common to let those experiences color the whole day. I work on switching that dynamic to recognize that the true beauty is in the contrast. *Most* of the time working with kids is really cool. It's the best job in the world, and even those less than stellar moments have something to teach us.

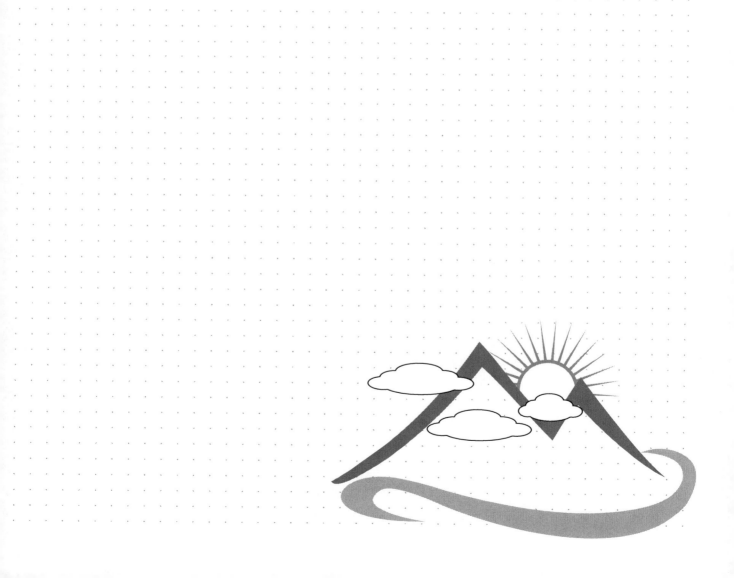

Practice 2 - Notice how small you are and how freeing that can be

I have been teaching for 23 years, so I've worked with over two thousand students. Obviously I can't remember all of them individually, but I love knowing that my presence in their lives might be a small contribution to the person they became. It's a little mind-boggling to think about 2000 adults out in the world who all had Mr. Smith as their English teacher. It makes me feel like a small cog in a much bigger machine.

Notice how small you are and how freeing that can be. I feel a similar sensation when I look at the night sky and contemplate the stars. We're so tiny, mere specks in the cosmic order, yet our actions can have ripples that extend without end. Observe nature whenever you have the chance and marvel at the interconnectedness of all things. Everything from the smallest insect to the largest mammal play their parts.

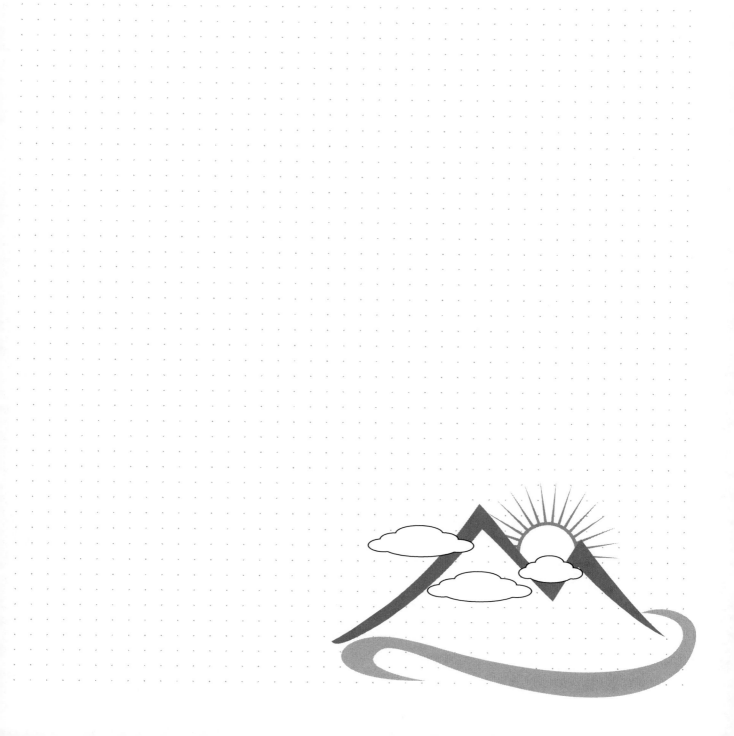

Practice 3 - Embrace the not knowing because some things are unknowable

There are some things that we just don't know, and maybe that's the point. I don't completely understand the science behind intermittent fasting. I respect the efforts of those who strive for that knowledge, but for me, the personal experiences I've had with fasting are enough. The human body is a complicated creation, and our understanding of how it works will probably continue to evolve for as long as we are on the planet. I'm OK with that.

Embrace the not knowing because some things are unknowable. The really big mysteries of life, the questions that people have been wrestling with for all of human history, will remain mysteries. Maybe the point is not to know all the answers, but to seek meaning while we're here and accept the uncertainty. I'm OK with that, too.

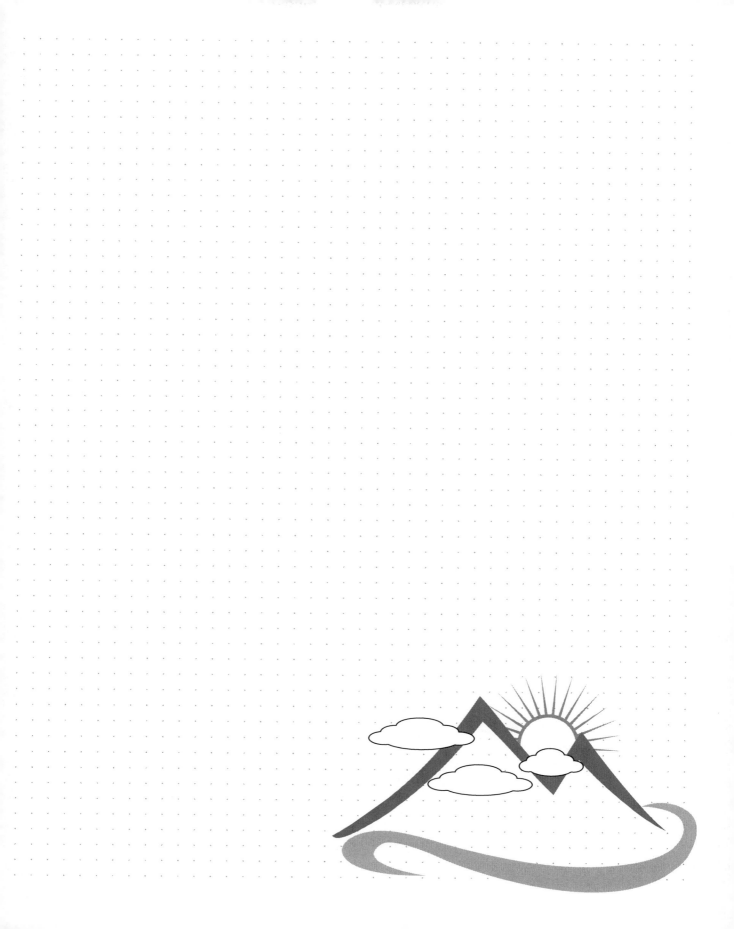

Process

▲ Do you have unrealistic expectations about how good or easy life is supposed to be?

▲ Do life's difficulties prevent you from seeing the positive things in your life?

▲ Have you considered the impact of your actions on others, in small ones and larger ones?

▲ What do you believe about your purpose?

▲ What gives you a sense of connection to something larger than yourself?

▲ Are you comfortable with the answers that you have now?

▲ Where are you in your own search for meaning?

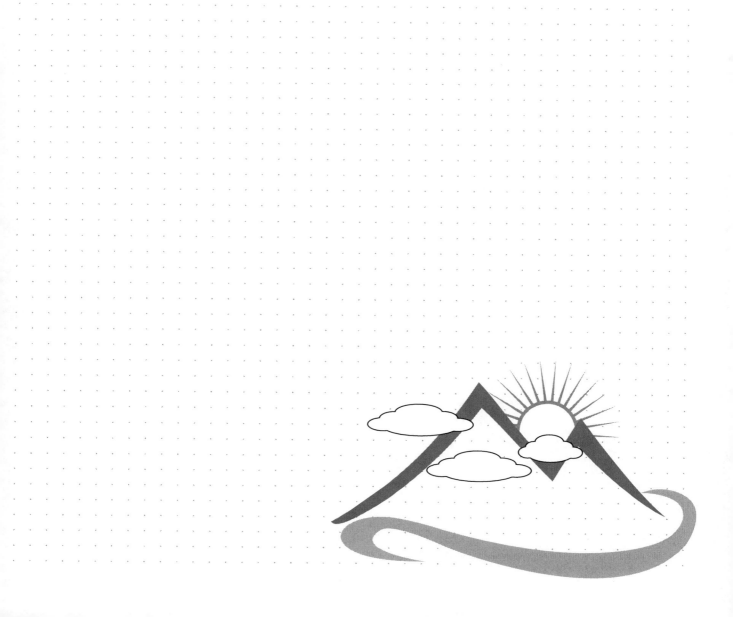

Conclusion

Thank you for reading *Fasting is the Foundation: A Real Man's View of Unbelievable Freedom.* I hope that my personal story inspires you in some small way to reflect on your own life and make positive change.

Unbelievable Freedom is not a destination, something you arrive at when you reach a number on the scale or achieve a particular physical feat. For me, it's a never-ending process of consciously evolving my mindset, letting go of the negative and embracing the positive. It's not linear or quick or easy. I'm not where I want to be yet, but I'm happier...and more free...than ever before.

Enjoy your journey.

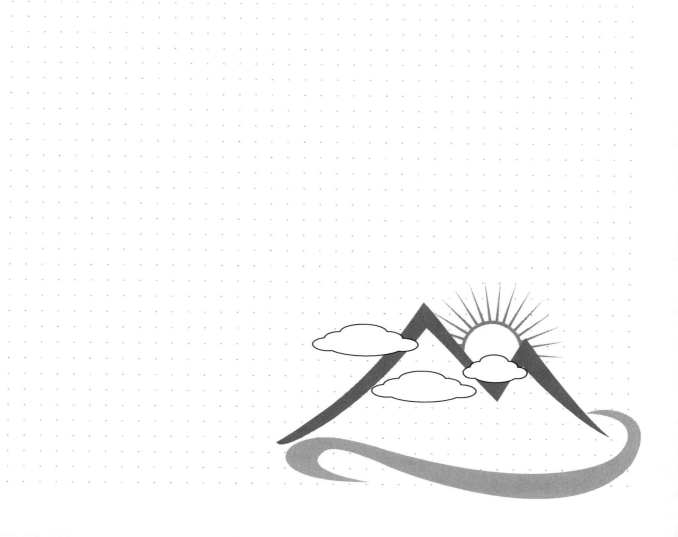

Continue The Journey With Ryan

Connect with Ryan through the following social media channels:

Unbelievable Freedom on Facebook

@unbelievablefreedom on Instagram

www.unbelievablefreedom.com

Or email ryan@unbelievablefreedom.com

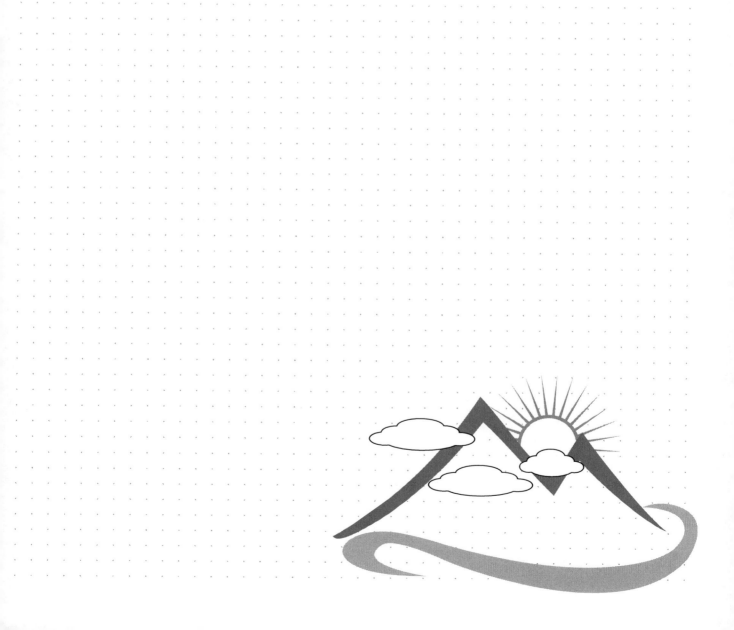

The Unbelievable Freedom Habit Guide Series

If you enjoyed this book and would like to continue your
Unbelievable Freedom journey, there are other titles to collect!

Fasting Feasting Freedom: A 33 Day Habit Creation Guide by Kim Smith

Poster Girl Habits: Creating an Intentional Contentment Practice by Kim Smith

A Superhero You: Activate Your Unstoppable Powers by Barbara Anne Cookson

Embracing Next: An Empty Nest Enjoyment Guide by Kim Smith

The Flow Lane: Creating Life One Thought At A Time by Lynn M Robinson

Script A New Life: A Guide to Lasting Change Creation by Tam Veilleux

Spark Your She: Radiance and Resilience in Your Season of Motherhood by Lindsay Harrington

Stop. Drop. Tap! Emotional Freedom Technique for Confidence & Clarity by Tam Veilleux

Information about all of these workbook-style Habit Guides
can be found at www.unbelievablefreedom.com,
along with links to their Amazon listings.

Believe in Unbelievable Freedom

Enjoy Your Life!

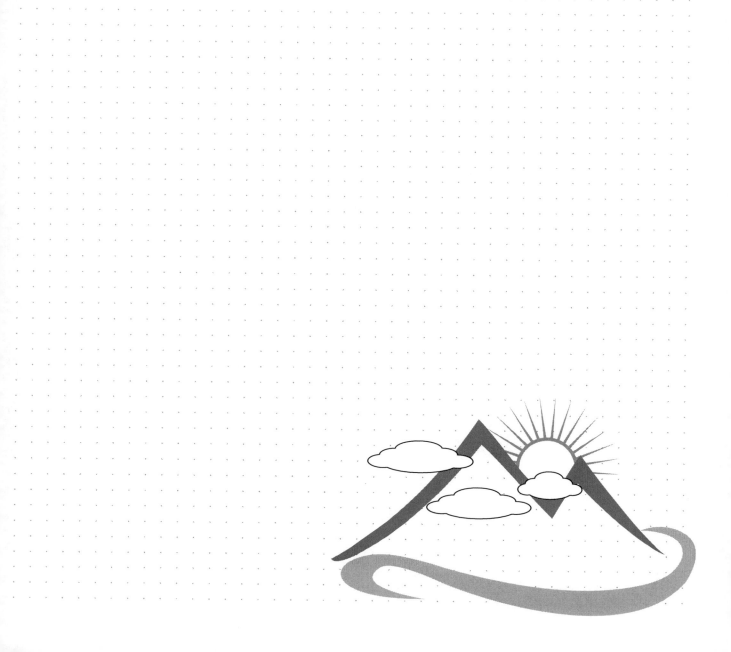

Made in the USA
Middletown, DE
03 April 2021

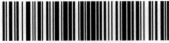